a guide to

essential oils

a guide to
essential oils

Jennie Harding

p

Designed and created with the Bridgewater Book Company Ltd.

NOTE

Any information given in this book is not intended to be taken as a
replacement for medical advice. Any person with a condition requiring
medical attention should consult a qualified medical practitioner or therapist.

WARNING

Never leave a burning candle unattended.

ACKNOWLEDGEMENTS

The publishers wish to thank the following for the use of pictures:

Art Directors and Trip: 12t, 20b, 23t, 29t, 32t, 48t, 49b; *A–Z Botanical
Collection Ltd*: 8b, 19t, 34t, 37t, 39t;
Corbis UK Ltd: 18b, 23b, 38, 53t;
Garden Picture Library: 47b; *Getty
Images*: 7t, 10t, 11t, 24t, 36b, 59b;
*Harry Smith Horticultural
Photographic Collection*: 33t.

contents

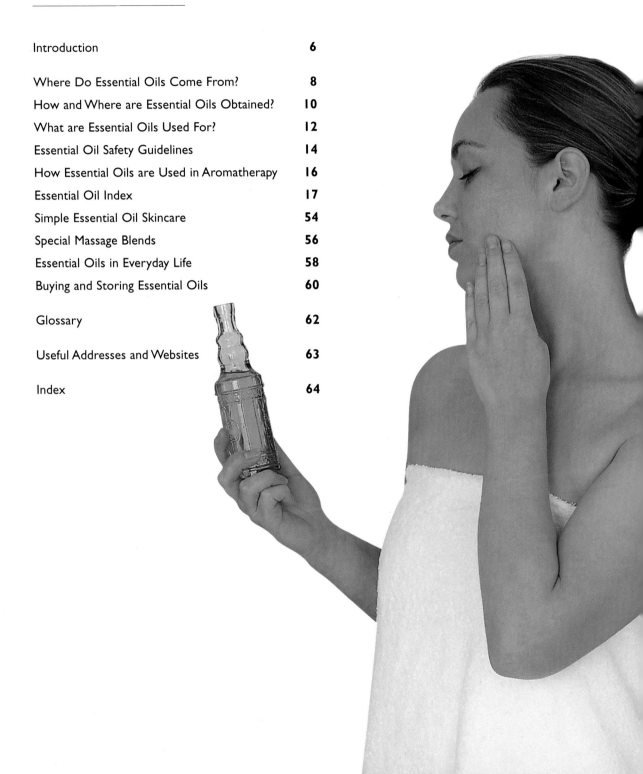

Introduction: What are Essential Oils?

Humans love aromatic plants. When we pass a beautiful, scented flower our behaviour shows this very clearly. The fragrance is enough to stop us in our tracks, make us forget our train of thought and plunge our face into the petals to inhale the perfume. When we do, we forget the cares and troubles of the day for a moment, and the world seems to be a simpler place. Gardeners love to touch and smell the herbs and aromatic grasses that they grow themselves, sniffing the aromas that cling to the fingers, such as pungent rosemary or zesty peppermint, fresh lavender or tangy fennel. These mouthwatering scents make us relax and breathe deeply.

All these perfumes we are inhaling and enjoying so enthusiastically are essential oils, the natural fragrances of aromatic plants. These scents are manufactured by the plants

Flowers attract our sense of smell like a magnet. We are drawn to plants such as scented roses.

The pungent herb rosemary uplifts the senses and excites the tastebuds. It is easily grown in a pot outside.

themselves and held in their tissues, only to be released through touch or the heat of the sun. Of all the plants on the Earth, only about one per cent contain essential oils. Humans have enjoyed a special relationship with these species since antiquity, and we have used such plants for perfumes, incense and medicines.

Aromatherapy relies on essential oils to achieve gentle, nurturing effects on body and mind. The oils are used on the skin, in the bath and through inhalation to promote relaxation

Relaxing in a bath with essential oils soothes the senses and can bring relief from aches and pains in the body.

and wellbeing. Essential oils and aromatherapy can make a very positive contribution to emotional and physical health, bringing a sense of inner peace and balance.

The Guide to Essential Oils takes you on an in-depth journey through the world of essential oils, where they come from and how they are obtained. It is an exploration of the particular plants that produce essential oils, revealing their unique role as a natural healing resource. The Essential Oils Index on pages 17–53 lists 36 common essential oils in detail, helping you get to know more about them and how to use them on yourself, friends and family. The methods are straightforward and easy to use in everyday situations. You will also find information about safety issues, buying and keeping the oils, and simple skincare routines.

You may well find that collecting essential oils, enjoying their aromas and learning about their different uses, becomes a fascinating pastime, something that develops from being a hobby into, quite simply, a way of life.

This book links the essential oils to the plants from which they are extracted. The botanical emphasis of this approach helps us to remember that all life on Earth is dependent on plants. As custodians of the planet we need to use these natural resources in a sustainable way if we are to continue to enjoy them.

Peppercorns yield a warming and stimulating essential oil that can ease painful joints and muscles.

Where Do Essential Oils Come From?

Essential oils are obtained from a small variety of aromatic plants. To understand essential oils, it helps to know something about how plants that provide essential oils function: through their roots, wood, leaves, flowers, fruits and seeds. Essential oils may be found in any of these plant parts.

The Magic of Plants

Plants are the most astonishing interactive energy systems, able to respond to the most minute changes in environmental conditions at all times during their life span. They are in the business of survival, competition and reproduction, and over millions of years they have evolved precise mechanisms to achieve this, of which essential oils are one. Botanists are unsure why particular plants have evolved to contain essential oils. However, here are some suggestions.

Essential oils are found in a variety of plant parts. The roots, wood, leaves, flowers, fruits and berries can all yield up their precious perfumes.

other insects. This helps to protect delicate root tissue from damage and allows maximum water uptake.

Roots

Roots draw minerals and water into the plant tissue as well as giving stability to the growing plant. Aromatic roots such as turmeric or vetiver, which grow in hot tropical locations, are unsavoury to invading grubs, beetles and

Wood

Trees like sandalwood or cedarwood contain essential oils in the heartwood of their trunks

Essential oils in leaves may have a protective function. This is the ylang ylang plant – the beautiful blooms nestle within the large dark-green leaves and are protected from the elements.

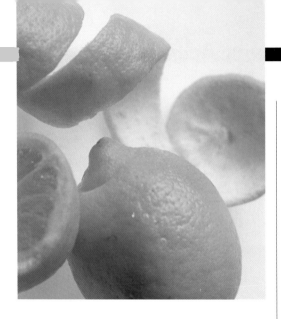

Essential oils that are found in the rind of fruits have a pungent and long-lasting aroma, making them popular scents.

and branches. There is some evidence that oils help to protect the inner structure of the wood from attack by beetles and other insects. Shrubs like frankincense and myrrh secrete resin, a sticky substance rich in essential oils, to protect themselves if their bark is cracked or damaged. The resin has been collected by humankind for thousands of years and burned as incense.

Leaves

In the leaves of any plant, the process of photosynthesis uses sunlight to convert carbon, hydrogen and oxygen to sugars. This process is vital for the growth of the plant, its eventual flowering and successful reproduction. Essential oils in the leaves may protect them from fungi or microbial attack, ensuring the maximum surface is available for the production of the plant's food.

Flowers

Some of the floral essential oils that are used in aromatherapy include subtle and exquisite fragrances such as lavender, rose, jasmine or orange blossom. The essential oils of other plants, such as frangipani, tuberose or mimosa, are very expensive to extract and are used in the formulation of some of the costliest perfumes. Flowers have only one purpose – to attract pollinating insects. The chemistry of attraction is a vital part of the insect–plant relationship. Some flowers have evolved aromas that mimic exactly the scent of specific insects. For example, the giant waterlily (*Victoria amazonica*) copies the pheromonal odour of a night-flying beetle, which has been pollinating the plant for centuries. Humans also have a long tradition of using the aroma of flowers to attract a mate – hence our love of perfumes.

Fruits and Seeds

Essential oils can be extracted from the rind of all citrus fruits. They are also found in the berries of bushes such as juniper. Fruits and berries are the end result of the flowering process. They tend to be aromatic in order to encourage animals or birds to eat them. The seeds are indigestible and are therefore excreted into the soil, giving the seed a better chance of germinating successfully.

How and Where are Essential Oils Obtained?

The production of essential oils involves a considerable investment of time, labour and skill. Plants are cultivated, harvested and processed to produce oils, which may then be shipped vast distances before reaching the consumer. Essential oils are a natural resource dependent on correct balances of soil composition, sun and rain to achieve good harvests year by year – just like any other natural crop.

Many essential oils are found in distant locations worldwide. Mediterranean plants need sunlight to develop properly.

Geography

Essential oils are found in different plant groups all over the world. One of the most common is the botanical family *Labiatae,* which includes many Mediterranean plants such as rosemary, marjoram and lavender. Most of the oils used in aromatherapy come from plants grown in southern Europe and North Africa, as these need a lot of sunlight to produce their oils. The same geographical region is the home of many citrus fruits in the *Rutaceae* family, including succulent oranges, lemons and mandarins, whose peel is full of essential oil.

Further afield you find the trees, flowers and spices of India, for example, producer of jasmine, sandalwood, cardamom and patchouli oils. Indonesia produces some of the more unusual oils, such as vetiver, which has a smoky, earthy aroma. The best geranium oil comes from the island of Réunion in the Indian Ocean, while Australia is the biggest producer of tea tree oil.

Cardamom pods produce a warm, fragrant and spicy essential oil.

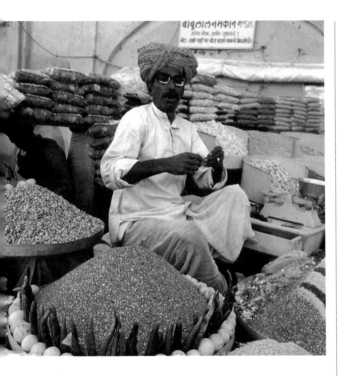

India is a huge producer of spices, aromatics and fragrances. Some of the more unusual oils come from this great continent.

When buying an oil, check the Essential Oil Index (see pages 17–53) to see where it is produced and just how far it has travelled!

Cultivation

The cultivation of essential oils requires a lot of land to produce bulk supplies of plants. For example, it takes approximately half a tonne of lavender material to produce just one litre of essential oil. Successful lavender farms need many hectares of land.

Oils like vetiver are produced in developing countries where farmers use high levels of manual labour and traditional techniques. Very often the labour lies in the collection process where plants cannot be harvested mechanically. In Bulgaria, roses are picked off the bush by hand – roughly 50–100 rose blooms are used for one drop of essential oil.

More mechanised essential oil cultivation is found in Australia, where tea tree oil is produced on a large scale on plantations using modern machinery for harvesting.

Extraction Methods

Essential oils are held in sacs or special microscopic cells within the plant tissues themselves. To extract the oil, different techniques are used:

Steam distillation passes steam at high pressure through the plant material, releasing the globules of essential oil into the water vapour. The fragrant steam is cooled back to water, and the essential oil can then be skimmed off as it floats on the surface. This technique is used to extract most oils, including lavender and rosemary.

Expression involves pressing the oil directly out of citrus fruit peel.

Solvent extraction uses chemical solvents to dissolve aromatic compounds out of delicate plant tissues. The extract is refined to produce an 'absolute'. Jasmine oil is produced by solvent extraction.

What are Essential Oils Used For?

In the last ten years, more and more people have been using essential oils and aromatherapy has become very popular. However, it may surprise you to discover that essential oils have a long history of use, both in aromatherapy and in other areas.

Ancient Egyptian men and women used aromatic fragrances to perfume the body and the hair.

Perfumery

Essential oils have been the basic ingredients in perfume formulae since the invention of a form of distillation by Avicenna, an Arab perfumer, mystic and herbalist, at the beginning of the last millennium. Even before that, essential oils were extracted by a method called enfleurage, in which aromatic plant material was pressed into trays of fat, which were then heated in an oven or left out in the sun. The melted fat was strained and then allowed to set, and the solid, scented 'unguent' used as a fragrance on the skin and hair.

In the past, only the most wealthy could afford the rare and costly extracts that were available. Perfumes were a sign of wealth and status. At the beginning of the twentieth century, the development of synthetic aromatic chemicals meant that perfume formulae could be copied, which is what happens in the mass production of fragrances today. Natural essential oils and aromatic extracts continue to be used for the creation of new formulae for perfumes, which are then synthetically reproduced.

Peppermint oil is used to flavour confectionery, including chocolates.

Food Flavouring

Many of the foodstuffs and drinks that we consume are flavoured with essential oils. Obvious examples include the use of peppermint and citrus oils in chocolate and other confectionery. However, many oils are used to give 'natural' flavours and fragrances to food products. They are used in preserved meats, alcoholic drinks, pickles and sauces. The amounts of essential oil used are very small and are carefully monitored to be at safe levels for internal consumption, because essential oils are extremely concentrated. In aromatherapy, essential oils are never swallowed. (See 'Essential Oil Safety Guidelines', pages 14–15.)

Pharmaceuticals

As well as being used in many foodstuffs, peppermint oil is used in pharmaceutical products such as toothpaste. Other essential oils that have pharmaceutical purposes include camphor and eucalyptus, which are used in commercial cough medicines, chest rubs and ointments for muscular aches and pains. Many of these products have been licensed since the early twentieth century.

Aromatherapy

Of all the tonnes of essential oils produced worldwide each year, only about five to ten per cent are used in aromatherapy. This is often a surprise to people, because they may be aware of essential oils only as the main ingredient in aromatherapy and not realise that they are so widely used elsewhere. In aromatherapy, it is very important that the oils used are totally natural and unadulterated with synthetics – trustworthy suppliers will buy directly from growers all around the world (for suppliers see page 61).

Essential oils such as that found in the citrus fruit orange are often used as food flavourings and preservatives.

Essential oils such as peppermint or fennel are used to flavour different kinds of toothpaste the world over.

Essential Oil Safety Guidelines

Essential oils are completely natural. However, it is important to be aware that they are highly concentrated and need to be used safely and correctly. These guidelines will help you to check how to use essential oils in particular situations. It is advisable to consult your medical practitioner if you have any physical or psychological symptoms, as essential oils are not a replacement for professional medical treatment.

No to Oral Use

The most important safety guideline is simply this: do not take essential oils by mouth. They are highly concentrated substances and in large amounts they can do internal damage. If oils have been swallowed accidentally, seek medical help immediately.

Pregnancy Care

If you are pregnant, lactating or breastfeeding, it is especially important not to swallow any essential oils. Any oils you use on yourself for massage or in the bath should be in very weak dilutions. If you are making any of the blends in this book, you should use half the

Women who are pregnant or breastfeeding need to be very careful when using essential oils.

stated number of drops. You are best advised to use flower and fruit oils only, as these are very gentle. It is a good idea to consult a qualified aromatherapist for advice.

Skin Safety

Before being applied to the skin, essential oils should always be diluted in a carrier oil such as sweet almond or grapeseed because they are so concentrated. Provided that you do not have sensitive skin (a tendency to allergic reactions), you can use lavender or tea tree neat for first aid purposes (two drops on a cotton bud applied to the affected area). If you are sensitive to nuts, it is best to avoid sweet almond oil and use grapeseed instead.

Phototoxic Oils

Essential oils from the citrus fruits – bergamot, grapefruit, orange, lemon, lime and mandarin – contain an ingredient that can cause skin

Only tea tree and lavender essential oils should be used neat on the skin. Other oils are not safe for such use.

reactions in sunlight. If you massage a blend with citrus oils into your skin, avoid direct exposure to strong UV light or a sunbed for 12 hours after application. This caution does not apply to inhalations or vaporisations with these oils.

High Blood Pressure

Rosemary essential oil is very stimulating and should be avoided if you have high blood pressure. Calming oils like lavender or ylang ylang are preferred for their soothing effects.

Epilepsy and Asthma

Again, rosemary essential oil has the potential to slightly increase the frequency of epileptic seizures, so it should be avoided by people who have epilepsy. Calming oils like sandalwood, neroli or orange are better suited for people with epilepsy. (Never attempt to apply oils during a seizure.) If you have asthma, it is advisable not to do inhalations with essential oils – use them for bathing, vaporisation and massage.

Babies and Children

Correct dosage of essential oils is especially crucial because of the delicate skin of small children. Follow these recommendations:

Babies up to 2 years: one drop of roman camomile **or** rose otto **or** lavender in 20 ml sweet almond carrier oil for general skin care and baby massage.

Children 2–10 years: any blends made from this book should contain half the stated number of drops. If an odd number of drops is given, reduce this to just under half (e.g. reduce 3 drops to 1, or 5 to 2).

Children over the age of 10: can receive oils in the same dilutions as adults.

Elderly Skin

In cases where the skin is delicate and very transparent with visible veins, you should use half the stated number of drops in any blend you make from this book so that the skin is nourished by the oils more gently.

Blends for children (and the elderly) contain low amounts of essential oils. Young skin is sensitive while older skin is more delicate.

How Essential Oils are Used in Aromatherapy

Aromatherapy is what it says it is – the 'aroma' being the fragrances of essential oils, and the 'therapy' the way in which the fragrance is applied to relieve physical symptoms and promote mental wellbeing. There are several simple ways to use essential oils, including in baths, inhalation and massage.

Baths

For a 20-minute soak to relieve tension and stress, run the bath to a comfortable temperature. Sprinkle 4 drops maximum of one essential oil or 3 drops each of two essential oils as a combination onto the surface of the water. Agitate the water gently to disperse the oils before getting in. If you have dry or sensitive skin, you can dilute the essential oils in 20 ml full-cream milk or unfragranced bath oil before adding them to the water. A simple relaxing combination is 3 drops each of lavender and sandalwood.

Inhalation

This method helps to relieve colds, influenza or sinus problems. You need a large bowl just over half full of nearly boiling water. Sprinkle 2 drops each of eucalyptus and tea tree onto the surface, then cover your head with a towel and inhale the aromatic steam for 15–20 minutes. Remove your glasses or contact lenses so they don't steam up or irritate the eyes.

Using steam inhalation can help to ease colds or blocked sinuses. Always be very careful when using boiling water.

Vaporisation

Vaporisers gently heat up to evaporate the essential oil and disperse its fragrance into a room. You can buy a ceramic burner with tea light candles or one of the many electric models available. You should follow the manufacturer's guidelines when using the oils though; generally 4 drops of one oil or 3 drops each of two as a combination will scent a room for up to two hours. You can use tea tree and lemon essential oils to remove unpleasant odours, or choose a favourite aroma to create an environment that suits your mood.

Choose the essential oil that meets your particular need, then blend with massage oil or use in an inhalation.

An electrically powered fragrance diffuser can help ease breathing problems and is safe to be left on.

Massage

When using essential oils for massage, they first need to be diluted in a carrier oil. These are vegetable oils such as grapeseed, sweet almond or jojoba. Most of the massage blends in this book are based on a formula of using 10 drops of essential oils in 20 ml (4 teaspoons) carrier oil. The mixture should be stored in a clean glass bottle. Shake the mixture before use. This is a suitable dilution for massage on most skins and is enough to massage a full body, not including the face. Sensitive, very young or elderly skin requires only 5 drops in 20 ml. (See pages 56–57 for Special Massage Blends.) Your blends will last for a maximum of four weeks. If you want to make larger quantities, simply take 40 ml base oil and double the drops of essential oils in the blend formula.

Essential Oil Index

In this section, you will find 36 essential oils grouped according to the plant parts that produce them. Each essential oil file contains key information and blends to try out yourself to help ease physical conditions and rebalance mental and emotional states.

Root Oils

The energy of these oils is generally stabilising and grounding to the body. Originally they protect and strengthen the plants that produce them.

Ginger
Zingiber officinale

Pungent ginger root yields a warming and spicy essential oil. It can improve energy levels.

Plant profile: ginger is a key ingredient in the recipes of India and China. It is also used in Traditional Chinese Medicine for digestion and circulation problems. Ginger roots are dried before distillation, which means that the essential oil smells less pungent than the freshly chopped root.

Ginger has been used for centuries in Traditional Chinese Medicine to treat the digestion and circulation.

Safety information: no issues.

Fragrance profile: ginger has a dry, musty aroma, which is sharper and spicier as it evaporates, leaving behind a lingering sweetness.

Main uses: eases indigestion; warms and soothes aches and pains in muscles; improves poor circulation; improves energy.

Suggested blends: for indigestion, add 2 drops peppermint, 3 drops ginger and 5 drops lemon to 20 ml of carrier oil and then massage into the abdomen gently.

Aches and pains can be eased by a taking a bath with 4 drops lavender and 2 drops ginger. Improve poor circulation by massaging a blend of 6 drops black pepper and 4 drops ginger in 20 ml carrier oil into the skin. You will notice the area becomes pink – this is an indication of improved circulation and is quite normal.

Vetiver is a very successful commercial crop in Indonesia as well as being a valuable essential oil.

Vetiver

Vetiveria zizanoides

Plant profile: vetiver comes mainly from Indonesia, where it is known locally as *akar wangi*. It is a tough tropical grass that is economically important to growers. The upper leaves can be woven into mats and fibres, while the aromatic roots are harvested for distillation. Vetiver is also grown on the island of Réunion in the Indian Ocean.

Safety information: no issues.

Fragrance profile: a very unusual deep, earthy, smoky aroma, heavy and warm.

Main uses: warms and relieves aches and pains, particularly backache; improves circulation; eases menstrual cramps; helps to ground and stabilise the emotions in cases of extreme stress.

Suggested blends: vetiver has a strong aroma, so no more than 2 drops are needed in a blend. For aches and pains and circulation, try 2 drops vetiver, 3 drops ginger and 5 drops lavender in 20 ml carrier oil for daily massage.

Menstrual cramps can be eased using a blend of 8 drops marjoram and 2 drops vetiver in 20 ml carrier oil, massaged over the lower abdomen twice daily.

Emotional insecurity can be calmed by taking a bath with 1 drop vetiver, 1 drop neroli and 3 drops lavender. You can also add these oils to 10 ml carrier oil and massage gently into the skin after your bath.

Massage an aching back with vetiver for relief from the pain. The warming scent is also very soothing to the mind and senses.

Angelica

Angelica archangelica

Plant profile: a herb that has been highly regarded in Western herbal tradition since medieval times; angelica is now cultivated for essential oil extraction in countries including Germany and Hungary. The whole plant is aromatic. It grows up to 2 metres in height and has dramatic spherical heads of tiny flowers. The pungent root has been used in herbal medicine for hundreds of years as a general cleanser and detoxifier.

Safety information: angelica essential oil is phototoxic. After any application to the skin, avoid direct exposure to strong sunlight or a sunbed for 12 hours. Angelica oil is best avoided in pregnancy.

The whole of the angelica plant is aromatic. However, it is the root of the plant that is used in the distillation of the essential oil.

Fragrance profile: sweet and aniseed-like, with a rich, warm and spicy note that is released as it evaporates.

Main uses: eases muscular aches, soothes arthritic joints and rheumatic pains; eases indigestion problems and wind and improves poor appetite; an overall energy tonic and revitaliser, especially in the springtime.

Suggested blends: for muscular aches and pains, add 2 drops angelica, 2 drops vetiver and 5 drops lavender to 20 ml carrier oil and apply using gentle massage.

Digestion problems can be eased by blending 3 drops peppermint, 4 drops ginger and 3 drops angelica in 20 ml carrier oil for massage over the abdomen.

A 'springtime blend' to help to energise and tone body and mind is 2 drops angelica, 3 drops juniper and 5 drops grapefruit in 20 ml carrier oil, to be massaged briskly into the skin after a bath or shower.

The angelica plant produces beautiful spherical flowerheads. These are made up of thousands of tiny flowers. Angelica is now specifically cultivated for essential oil extraction.

Turmeric

Curcuma longa/Curcuma domestica

Yellow turmeric roots have many uses – they can be used as a cooking spice or an essential oil.

Plant profile: turmeric is a plant that looks very like ginger, with tall shoots and abundant elegant leaves, and is a member of the same botanical family. The highly aromatic roots are bright yellow and are used to colour curries. The roots are cleaned and sun-dried before being ground as a spice or distilled for the oil. India, China and Indonesia are the main producers.

Safety information: no issues.

Fragrance profile: dry, musty and vegetable-like aroma; spicy and sweet as it evaporates.

Main uses: soothes and eases backache and muscular pains; improves circulation; tones and improves the digestion, easing stomach cramps and constipation. Very stabilising and grounding to overwrought emotions; warms and re-energises the body.

Suggested blends: for aches and pains, add 4 drops turmeric, 4 drops ginger and 2 drops vetiver to 20 ml carrier oil and massage the affected areas gently.

Cramps and indigestion can be eased by blending 4 drops turmeric, 2 drops lemongrass and 4 drops ginger in 20 ml carrier oil, and massaging the blend into the abdomen.

For emotional tension, add 1 drop turmeric, 2 drops neroli and 2 drops ginger to a warm bath and rest there for 20 minutes.

This combination can also be added to 10 ml carrier oil and massaged into the skin afterwards.

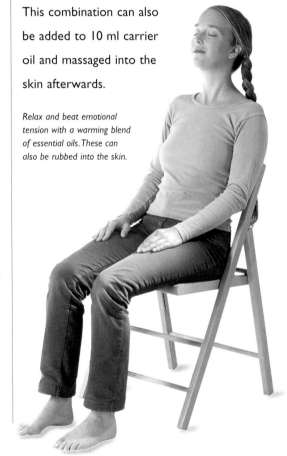

Relax and beat emotional tension with a warming blend of essential oils. These can also be rubbed into the skin.

Wood Oils

These oils are found in the aromatic heartwood in the centre of tree trunks and branches. They are at the centre of the growing, spreading height of the tree. The energy of these oils is more expansive, encouraging deep breathing.

Sandalwood
Santalum album

Plant profile: the best-quality sandalwood comes from the Mysore region of India near Bangalore. It takes approximately 30 years for the wood to mature to its full aromatic potential, so planting and harvesting is carefully rotated and controlled. The wood is used in the distillation of sandalwood oil. It is also powdered for making incense sticks and cosmetics, and can be carved into statues and boxes.

Safety information: no issues.

Fragrance profile: this beautiful oil should be thick and pale golden, with a subtle aroma at first, deepening to a rich, woody, spicy, sweet fragrance as it evaporates.

Main uses: eases tight chesty coughs, colds, sore throats; soothes dry chapped skin and improves the texture of all skin types; eases depression, anxiety and feelings of panic.

Suggested blends: for coughs, add 3 drops sandalwood, 3 drops cedarwood and 4 drops lemon to 20 ml carrier oil and massage gently over the chest area.

A rejuvenating skincare blend is 6 drops sandalwood, 2 drops patchouli and 2 drops rose in 20 ml jojoba oil, massaged into the face at night.

To ease anxiety or depression, add 3 drops sandalwood and 2 drops orange to a warm bath and rest for 20 minutes. Add the same oils to 10 ml carrier oil and massage into the skin afterwards.

Sandalwood brings a state of peace and calm to body and mind. It is also good for use on sensitive skins.

Atlas Cedarwood

Cedrus atlantica

Plant profile: these tall, majestic cedar trees come from the Atlas mountains in Morocco. They stand over 30 metres in height with a sweeping, tentlike appearance, and a wonderful aroma floats around them thanks to the essential oil in the red heartwood. Cedar was used extensively by the ancient Egyptians in the manufacture of furniture and ships because of the wood's resistance to insects – as well as its beauty.

Safety information: no issues.

Fragrance profile: sharp and fresh with a sweet, woody, soft undertone.

The ancient Egyptians used fragrant cedarwood to make beautiful and aromatic furniture.

Cedarwood trees are huge and majestic, and are wonderfully aromatic too. The oil comes from the red heartwood.

Main uses: eases bronchitis, chest infections, coughs; soothes cracked skin, eczema, acne and oily skin; assuages feelings of panic, calms and deepens the breath when under stress.

Suggested blends: for chest problems, add 3 drops cedarwood, 3 drops sandalwood and 4 drops lemon to 20 ml carrier oil and massage the chest. For cracked skin, try a blend of 3 drops cedarwood, 2 drops frankincense and 5 drops lavender in 20 ml carrier oil. For acne or oily skin, try 3 drops cedarwood, 2 drops tea tree and 5 drops lavender in 20 ml jojoba as a cleanser. For stress, vaporise 2 drops cedarwood and 3 drops lavender. Use these oils in 10 ml carrier oil to massage the neck and shoulders.

Resin Oils

These sticky aromatic substances, the original incense ingredients, ooze out of the bark of certain trees and shrubs as a defence against injury. We too can use them to heal our skin.

Frankincense
Boswellia carterii var. thurifera

Frankincense is the original 'true incense' of antiquity and has been burned in places of religious worship for centuries.

Plant profile: frankincense is a robust desert shrub with delicate leaves and whitish papery bark. The name actually means 'true incense', and it has been burned in religious ceremonies since ancient times. The frankincense plantations of the pharaohs were seen as one of the most valuable commodities in Egypt and frankincense was used in the embalming process. Cuts were made in the bark to make the gum ooze out. It is still used for incense and distilled for the oil, mainly in Somalia and Oman.

Safety information: no issues.

Frankincense gum forms 'tears' or granules. This oozes out of the bark of the frankincense shrub when it is cut.

Fragrance profile: fresh and sharp initially, deepening to woody, resiny with sweet notes.

Main uses: disinfects and heals cuts, wounds, eczema and damaged skin; tones and rejuvenates all skin types, especially mature; eases chesty coughs or bronchitis; comforts anxiety and emotional stress.

Suggested blends: a good skin-healing blend is 4 drops frankincense, 2 drops lavender and 4 drops cedarwood in 20 ml carrier oil. Apply to the affected area twice daily. A tonic for mature skin is 4 drops frankincense, 3 drops neroli and 3 drops rose in 20 ml jojoba oil. For chesty coughs, try an inhalation of 3 drops frankincense and 3 drops cedarwood. To ease emotional stress and help you relax, vaporise 3 drops frankincense and 4 drops grapefruit.

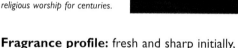

Myrrh

Commiphora myrrha

Plant profile: a thorny shrub, native to the arid climates of Somalia and Arabia, with papery bark and a reddish gum that oozes out when the bark is cracked or cut deliberately. Myrrh is soluble in water and has been used as a tonic for the teeth and gums since the time of Hippocrates (469–399 BCE), the father of Western medicine. Like frankincense, myrrh is prized for wound healing, and was used by the ancient Egyptians for embalming.

Myrrh gum is reddish-orange in colour and was used in the embalming process in ancient Egypt.

Safety information: myrrh is best avoided during pregnancy.

Fragrance profile: a dry, sharp and subtle aroma, which gradually deepens to reveal rich, sweet and spicy notes.

Main uses: heals and disinfects deep cuts, wounds, chapped and cracked skin, eczema; cleans and disinfects the mouth, easing sore gums and mouth ulcers; relieves bronchitis, chesty coughs; comforts and calms highly anxious emotional states.

Suggested blends: to help damaged skin, blend 3 drops myrrh, 4 drops tea tree and 3 drops frankincense in 20 ml carrier oil and apply 2–3 times daily. For problems in the mouth, add 2 drops myrrh to a glass of water, stir vigorously and use as a mouthwash (do not swallow). For chesty coughs, add 3 drops myrrh, 3 drops frankincense and 4 drops cedarwood to 20 ml carrier oil and massage chest area especially at night. To de-stress, add 2 drops myrrh and 3 drops geranium to a bath – and relax.

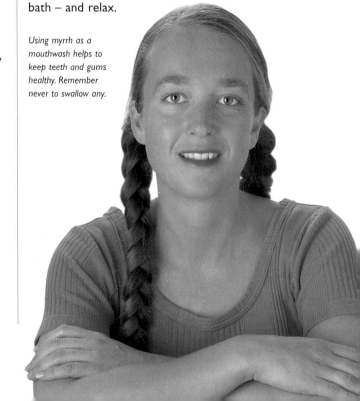

Using myrrh as a mouthwash helps to keep teeth and gums healthy. Remember never to swallow any.

Leaf Oils

These oils are contained in the all-important leaves that manufacture the plant's food. They protect the leaf surface from damage by fungi and bacteria.

Marjoram
Origanum marjorana

French marjoram has a gentle woody aroma. The scent evaporates quite quickly.

Plant profile: this is the species otherwise known as 'French marjoram', and not Spanish marjoram, which is a type of thyme. French marjoram has been a favourite herb for cooking and has been widely used for centuries. It is low-growing, with small aromatic leaves and tiny white flowers that appear in summer. Originally from Mediterranean regions, it will grow well in more northerly climates if kept sheltered and in a sunny spot. The essential oil comes from France.

Safety information: no issues.

Fragrance profile: a warm, woody aroma that somewhat resembles camphor, gradually becoming sweet and soft.

Main uses: helps muscular aches and pains, stiffness and strains; eases menstrual cramps and mood swings; helps migraine, headaches and nervous tension.

Suggested blends: for muscular aches, add 4 drops marjoram, 4 drops ginger and 2 drops vetiver to 20 ml carrier oil for massage. Menstrual symptoms can be eased by massaging the abdomen with 4 drops marjoram, 4 drops lavender and 2 drops vetiver in 20 ml oil.

For headaches and nervous tension, add 4 drops marjoram, 2 drops peppermint and 4 drops lavender to 20 ml carrier oil and gently massage the forehead, neck and shoulders.

Using essential oils like marjoram can help headaches and menstrual problems.

Peppermint

Mentha piperita

Peppermint is a strongly scented herb and grows very easily and quickly in the garden.

Plant profile: peppermint is a tall vigorous mint with a very invasive habit – ask any gardener! It spreads rapidly through tough root systems, and will displace other more tender herbs in a plot unless it is contained in some way. The square, erect stems support deep-green aromatic leaves and, if left untrimmed the plant will produce tall heads of tiny white flowers. Peppermint essential oil comes mostly from the USA, where it is used to flavour toothpaste and chewing gum.

Safety information: if your skin is sensitive, use half the stated drops of peppermint in any blend due to the menthol content in the oil, which can act as an irritant.

Fragrance profile: pungent, fresh, zesty and minty aroma with sweeter notes later.

Main uses: eases stomach cramps, indigestion, constipation and nausea; helps muscular aches, stiffness, backache; eases headaches and migraine; clears the head and improves concentration.

Suggested blends:

indigestion symptoms can be helped by massaging the abdomen with 2 drops peppermint, 4 drops ginger and 4 drops cardamom in 20 ml carrier oil.

For aches and pains, massage daily with 2 drops peppermint, 4 drops rosemary and 4 drops black pepper in 20 ml carrier oil. To ease headaches, add 2 drops peppermint and 3 drops lavender to 10 ml carrier oil and massage onto the forehead and neck.

For clearing the mind, vaporise 2 drops peppermint and 3 drops lemon.

Vaporising peppermint essential oil in the office can clear your head and kick-start the mind.

Rosemary

Rosmarinus officinalis

Rosemary is an evergreen herb with a bracing aroma. It is used in cooking as well as aromatherapy.

Plant profile: the name 'rosemary' means 'rose of the sea', a reference to the original habitat of the plant on the dry, sandy coastline of the Mediterranean Sea. Even today, the best pungent oil comes from Spain or North Africa; the hotter and dryer the climate, the better the aroma. Rosemary oil smells quite similar to eucalyptus because they have a fragrant ingredient in common: eucalyptol.

Safety information: rosemary is not advised for people with high blood pressure, as it is a stimulating oil. It should also be avoided by people who suffer from epilepsy.

Fragrance profile: strong, camphoraceous, fresh and herbal aroma with a definite eucalyptus tone.

Main uses: eases muscular aches and pains, backache, poor circulation; stimulates the scalp and eases dandruff; clears the breathing in colds, influenza or sinusitis; stimulates the mind and wakes up the brain.

Suggested blends: for aches and pains and for poor circulation, try using 4 drops rosemary, 2 drops lemongrass and 4 drops nutmeg in 20 ml carrier oil.

For a hair and scalp tonic, try adding 5 drops rosemary and 5 drops tea tree to 20 ml of unfragranced shampoo and then washing your hair as normal.

For easier breathing when suffering from colds or influenza, add 3 drops rosemary and 3 drops tea tree to a bowl of nearly boiling water and inhale the vapour for 20 minutes. To help stimulate the mind, vaporise 3 drops rosemary and 3 drops peppermint.

Rosemary oil improves concentration and sharpens the mind. It is useful in the workplace.

Cypress

Cupressus sempervirens

Plant profile: tall, evergreen cypress trees are an elegant feature of the landscape in Italy, France, Corsica, Sardinia, Spain and Portugal. The Latin name *sempervirens* means 'ever living', a reference to the long life of the species. They are often planted near dwellings or near churches to signify eternal life. The oil comes from the young twigs and leaves, which are highly aromatic. Distillation takes place mostly in France or Spain.

Safety information: no issues.

Fragrance profile: earthy, smoky and green with camphoraceous and sweet notes.

Main uses: clears oily skin and blocked pores; improves lymphatic drainage and cellulite; eases spasmodic coughs and bronchitis; soothes fraught emotions.

The tall dark shapes of cypress trees stand out clearly in a Mediterranean landscape.

Suggested blends: oily skin can be treated daily using 3 drops cypress, 3 drops tea tree and 4 drops grapefruit in 20 ml jojoba oil to cleanse and soothe the skin.

To counter cellulite, try using 4 drops cypress, 4 drops grapefruit and 2 drops juniper in 20 ml carrier oil for a vigorous daily massage of the affected areas.

To ease spasmodic coughs, do an inhalation with 3 drops cypress and 2 drops cedarwood twice daily; these oils can also be added to 10 ml carrier oil and massaged into the chest.

If your emotions are overstretched or you are suffering from stress, try taking a soothing bath with 3 drops cypress and 3 drops lavender and relax deeply.

Cypress essential oil is useful as a soothing skin treatment for an oily or blemished complexion.

Petitgrain (orange leaf)

Citrus aurantium var. *amara*

Petitgrain is one of three oils taken from the bitter orange tree. Unlike most citrus oils, petitgrain is not phototoxic.

Plant profile: petitgrain is one of the essential oils produced by the bitter orange tree. The other oils are neroli (orange blossom) and bitter orange oil (expressed from the rind of the fruit). The leaves of the orange tree contain tiny sacs of essential oil, which are visible (like grains) to the naked eye when a leaf is held up to the sun – the French name of the oil means 'little grain'. The oil is an original ingredient of eau de cologne, popular since the eighteenth century. Most petitgrain oil comes from France or Paraguay.

Safety information: no issues. (Unlike orange, this oil is not phototoxic.)

Fragrance profile: a green, fresh, bittersweet aroma with a hint of citrus.

Main uses: tones, refreshes and balances oily and combination skins; eases stomach cramps, indigestion and wind; calms and soothes the mind, releasing tension and nervous exhaustion.

Suggested blends: for oily/combination skin, add 4 drops petitgrain, 2 drops patchouli and 4 drops lavender to 20 ml jojoba oil and use as a cleanser and skin-soother twice a day.

To ease stomach cramps, add 4 drops petitgrain, 2 drops peppermint and 4 drops roman camomile to 20 ml carrier oil and massage the abdomen (half the dose of drops in 20 ml carrier can be used on children).

To relieve stress and calm the nerves, add 3 drops petitgrain and 3 drops sandalwood to a warm bath and relax.

Petitgrain is a fragrance note that can be found in many old-fashioned colognes.

Patchouli

Pogostemon patchouli

Patchouli leaves are soft, velvety and highly aromatic. The leaves are used in India to protect textiles from moths.

Plant profile: patchouli comes from India in the form of a thick, golden-brown essential oil with a very pronounced aroma. The leaves of the patchouli plant have a velvety texture thanks to thousands of tiny hairs on the surface. These contain microscopic sacs of essential oil, so that when you rub the leaf, the aroma is very strong on your fingers. Patchouli leaves are used to protect cloth from moths in India, and the oil is regarded as an insect repellent. It is also traditionally used in India as a skin conditioner and antiseptic.

Safety information: no issues.

Fragrance profile: a rich, velvety, musky aroma that develops spicy, earthy and sweet tones with time.

Main uses: helps to soothe cracked, chapped and dry skin and eczema; improves the complexion of mature and dry skins; increases sexual energy and helps to enhance sensuality.

Suggested blends: for dry, damaged or cracked skin, try creating a massage blend of 3 drops patchouli, 3 drops cedarwood and 4 drops roman camomile in 20 ml jojoba oil and apply to the area as needed.

To improve the complexion, try adding 3 drops patchouli, 4 drops frankincense and 3 drops sandalwood to 20 ml carrier oil and massage gently into the face, especially at night (this blend is appropriate for men and women).

For a sensual massage, blend add 3 drops patchouli, 2 drops rose and 5 drops orange to 20 ml carrier oil.

Patchouli makes a wonderful relaxing and sensual blend. The essential oil can increase and enhance sexual energy.

Eucalyptus
Eucalyptus globulus

Plant profile: there are more than 700 species of eucalyptus. In aromatherapy, several eucalyptus oils are used, of which *Eucalyptus globulus* is the most common. This evergreen tree from Australia can grow to a height of up to 90 metres when mature. The aromatic leaves are bluish-green on the upper surface and paler underneath. The leaves and the essential oil have been widely used as a household remedy in Australia from the days of the Aborigines in the treatment of fevers, respiratory conditions and skin infections.

Safety information: must not be swallowed – some cases of severe internal poisoning have occurred. Safe on the skin or as an inhalation.

The eucalyptus tree is native to Australia and is an attractive evergreen with blue-green foliage.

Fragrance profile: extremely fresh and bracing, with woodier tones later.

Main uses: clears colds, blocked noses, sinusitis, chest infections; soothes burns, cuts, wounds and insect bites; eases muscular pains; improves circulation; improves concentration.

Suggested blends: for colds and chest problems, use 2 drops eucalyptus and 3 drops tea tree in an inhalation twice daily. Add the same combination of oils to 10 ml carrier oil and massage into the chest area.

For damaged skin, add 2 drops eucalyptus, 3 drops tea tree and 5 drops lavender to 20 ml carrier oil and apply twice daily.

For muscle pains, add 3 drops eucalyptus, 4 drops rosemary and 3 drops ginger to 20 ml carrier oil for massage.

To help improve levels of concentration, vaporise 3 drops eucalyptus and 3 drops rosemary.

Eucalyptus is one of the best oils to use for inhalations and for clearing catarrh.

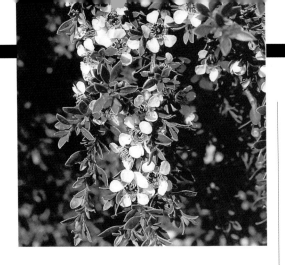

Tea tree essential oil is taken from the leaves of the tree and is very pungent and antiseptic.

Tea Tree

Melaleuca alternifolia

Plant profile: tea tree is native to Australia, where it has long been used by the aboriginal people as an antiseptic. The name 'tea tree' refers to the practice of drinking an infusion of the leaves as a healing herbal drink, first observed by the sailors on Captain Cook's ship in the eighteenth century. Production of the oil is now a huge commercial enterprise with a whole host of tea tree products available on the market, from toothpaste to foot powder. It is one of the most antiseptic plants ever discovered.

Tea tree can help to treat the symptoms of influenza. Inhale the oil from a tissue whenever necessary.

Safety information: safe to use neat on the skin (2 drops on a cotton wool pad applied directly to the affected area) except on individuals with sensitive or allergy-prone skin, for whom it must be diluted in carrier oil.

Fragrance profile: medicinal, green, camphoraceous aroma, pungent and strong.

Main uses: clears skin infections and acne; heals wounds and cuts; soothes insect bites; clears athlete's foot; helps influenza, colds, bronchitis; boosts general immunity.

Suggested blends: for skin infections, add 4 drops tea tree, 3 drops sandalwood and 3 drops lavender to 20 ml carrier oil and apply as necessary. To assist chest problems, use an inhalation of 3 drops tea tree and 3 drops lemon twice daily. To boost immunity, add 2 drops tea tree, 2 drops bergamot and 1 drop black pepper to a warm bath. Add this combination of oils to 10 ml carrier oil and massage the upper chest area. Do this daily during an episode of influenza.

Lemongrass
Cymbopogon citratus

Plant profile: lemongrass is an aromatic tropical grass from India. It is well known as a flavouring ingredient in Indian and Thai cooking. In India, the grass is used in traditional medicine to help reduce fevers and kill infections, and also as an insect repellent. The leaves are chopped just above ground level and, as with all grasses, new shoots are then produced very quickly.

Safety information: the oil is regarded as a potential irritant to already sensitive or allergic skin and is not advised for infants and young children. It should always be diluted in a carrier, even in bath blends.

Fragrance profile: a very strong, 'lemon sherbert' aroma that is zesty and sweet with a slightly heavy undertone.

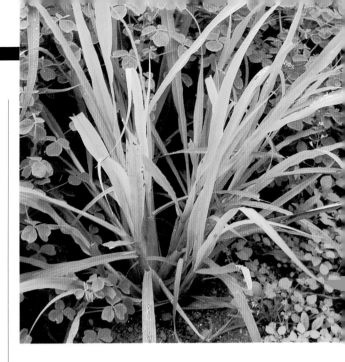

Lemongrass is a vigorous and aromatic tropical plant. It should always be diluted — even in blends for the bath.

Main uses: eases muscular aches, pains and stiffness; eases stomach cramps, indigestion and constipation; lifts depression or anxiety and improves the mood.

Suggested blends: for muscular aches, add 2 drops lemongrass, 3 drops rosemary and 5 drops cardamom to 20 ml carrier oil to massage the specific areas.

To ease stomach cramps or constipation, add 2 drops lemongrass, 4 drops coriander and 4 drops nutmeg to 20 ml carrier oil and massage the abdomen twice daily.

To improve mood and combat stress, add 2 drops lemongrass, 2 drops rose and 6 drops frankincense to 20 ml carrier oil.

Lemongrass is a key flavouring in most Thai dishes. Its zesty character can really lift a dish.

Palmarosa

Cymbopogon martini

Aromatic palmarosa is another grass grown in India. It has a similar fragrance to rose oil.

Plant profile: palmarosa is another aromatic grass from India, this time with a sweet smell and an altogether milder effect when used. In the past, it has often been used to adulterate or dilute pure rose oil, because the fragrance is somewhat similar and the grass is produced much more cheaply and in far larger quantities than rose. Palmarosa has a long-lasting aroma, which makes it a popular cosmetic ingredient in soaps, toiletries and perfumes.

Safety information: no issues.

Fragrance profile: a long-lasting, sweet and roselike aroma, which is soft and gentle with slightly lemony tones.

Main uses: soothes and calms irritated skin, acne, eczema, dermatitis; improves the facial complexion in all skin types, especially combination and mature; soothes cystitis and clears urinary tract infections; calms and de-stresses the nerves.

Suggested blends: for sensitive or irritated skin, add 3 drops palmarosa and 2 drops roman camomile to 20 ml carrier oil (note the low dilution) and apply as needed. To balance and rejuvenate the complexion, add 4 drops palmarosa, 3 drops frankincense and 3 drops sandalwood to 20 ml carrier oil and massage the face, especially at night. For cystitis or urinary problems, add 3 drops palmarosa and 3 drops sandalwood to a warm bath to soothe the area. To uplift your mood, add 3 drops palmarosa, 4 drops grapefruit and 3 drops orange to 20 ml carrier oil for an exotic and soft massage blend.

Palmarosa oil cares for and nurtures all skin types. It also de-stresses overstretched nerves.

Flower Oils

These are some of the most exquisite fragrances you will encounter. Captured from the petals, they are the unique aromatic signal of that plant.

Lavender

Lavandula angustifolia

Plant profile: lavender oil is now widely produced in the UK, southern France, Tasmania, New Zealand and Bulgaria. Purple lavender fields make one of the most wonderful aromatic landscapes, filled with bees and butterflies busily enjoying the magnificent supply of pollen. Lavender oils vary in fragrance according to the altitude where they are produced – high altitude oils have sharper and fresher aromas, and low altitude ones are sweeter and softer.

Safety information: no issues. Lavender can be used neat (2 drops on a cotton wool pad applied directly to the affected area).

Fragrance profile: mainly soft, sweet and floral with camphoraceous and pungent notes.

Main uses: soothes cuts, burns, wounds, insect bites, sore skin; eases headaches, migraine and muscular aches and tension; soothes chesty spasmodic coughs; helps insomnia, nervous tension and anxiety; useful for both adults and children.

Suggested blends: for skin problems, add 4 drops lavender, 3 drops tea tree and 3 drops roman camomile to 20 ml carrier oil and massage gently into the affected area.

Ease headaches by adding 3 drops lavender to 5 ml carrier oil and massaging the forehead and neck to provide relief.

To relieve coughs, an inhalation with 4 drops lavender and 3 drops cedarwood done twice daily can often be helpful.

To ease insomnia, vaporise 3 drops lavender and 3 drops orange to help you fall asleep.

Lavender fields are vibrantly purple and wonderfully aromatic. Bees and butterflies love visiting the plants that grow here.

Geranium

Pelargonium graveolens

The leaves of this geranium release a strong rosy aroma.

Plant profile:

this is a tropical geranium with velvety, frilly leaves. Rubbing the tiny surface hairs releases a strong, rosy aroma onto your fingers. The geranium grows as a shrub up to 1 metre in height and has pinkish flowers. The essential oil has a powerful floral aroma. The island of Réunion in the Indian Ocean produces the best-quality essential oil. Chinese and Egyptian geranium oils are also available but have a much heavier fragrance.

Safety information:

no issues.

Fragrance profile:

rosy, sweet and strong, with a hint of lemon and fresh green notes.

Main uses: soothes cracked and inflamed skin, eczema, dermatitis, acne and congested or oily skin; eases premenstrual symptoms such as lack of energy, bloatedness and fluid retention; soothes mood swings and helps to balance hormonally related emotional upsets.

Suggested blends: for skin problems, add 3 drops geranium, 3 drops sandalwood and 4 drops lavender to 20 ml carrier oil and apply to the area as needed.

To ease premenstrual symptoms, try adding 2 drops geranium and 3 drops petitgrain to a warm bath. You can also use the same combination of oils in 10 ml carrier oil for an uplifting massage afterwards.

To help balance mood swings, add 3 drops geranium, 3 drops lemon and 4 drops orange to 20 ml carrier oil and massage into your skin. This will give you a floral and citrus uplift.

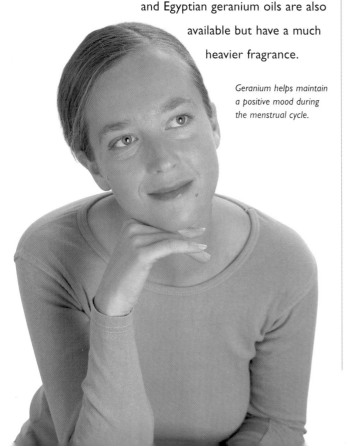

Geranium helps maintain a positive mood during the menstrual cycle.

Ylang Ylang

Cananga odorata

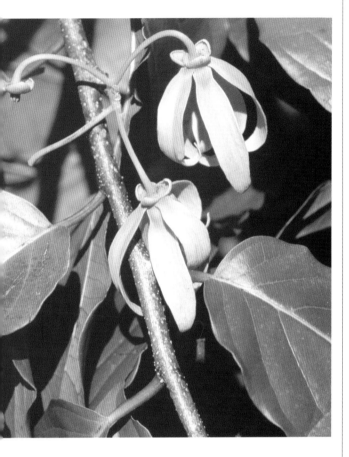

Ylang ylang flowers are beautiful exotic blooms, which yield large amounts of deeply scented essential oil.

Plant profile: all the way from Madagascar, a magical island off the coast of East Africa, comes the 'flower of flowers' – ylang ylang. Beautiful, lush, golden-yellow flowers with velvety petals produce a wonderful oil with a strong resemblance to jasmine. There is such a high content of fragrance in the flowers that the essential oil can be drawn off three times during the process of distillation, giving rise to three grades of essential oil. The first collection of oil is known as the 'perfume' grade and is the best quality.

Safety information: no major issues. Some individuals find the strong floral aroma brings on a headache.

Fragrance profile: sharp and sweet, becoming deeply floral, jasmine-like, heady and soft with time.

Main uses: tones oily and combination skins; reduces panic attacks and stress-related anxiety symptoms; soothes and calms emotional stress and overstretched nerves.

Suggested blends: to tone oily skin, add 2 drops ylang ylang, 3 drops sandalwood and 5 drops frankincense to 20 ml jojoba oil and use as a cleanser and skin-soother twice daily.

For panic and anxiety attacks, add 2 drops ylang ylang and 3 drops lavender to a warm bath, and add the same combination of oils to 10 ml carrier oil for a relaxing neck and shoulder massage afterwards.

To soothe the nerves and ease anxiety, add 2 drops ylang ylang, 2 drops patchouli and 5 drops orange to 20 ml carrier oil and massage your body gently.

Rose

Rosa damascena

Plant profile: costly and labour-intensive to produce, rose is one of the most beautiful of all essential oils. The little damask rose from Kazanlik in Bulgaria produces the finest quality rose oil, although Turkish, Moroccan and Russian rose oils are also excellent. Rose 'otto' is simply distilled rose oil – between 50 and 100 blooms are needed per drop. An 'absolute' of rose, chemically extracted, is also available at a slightly lower cost. Look out for pure rose oil already diluted in jojoba as a more affordable and still effective way to use this oil.

Safety information: no issues.

Fragrance profile: honey-sweet, slightly lemony and soft, with richness and depth.

The damask rose has a uniquely glorious aroma. It is one of the most costly oils to produce but is worth every drop.

Main uses: tones and rejuvenates all skin types, especially dry, sensitive and mature; eases premenstrual and menopausal symptoms; helps release feelings of grief and separation, restoring the heart.

Suggested blends: to tone the skin, add 2 drops rose, 4 drops frankincense and 4 drops sandalwood to 20 ml jojoba oil (halve the number of drops for sensitive skin).

To help relieve premenstrual or menopausal symptoms, add 4 drops rose, 3 drops neroli and 3 drops mandarin to 20 ml carrier oil and massage into the body.

To ease grief, add 2 drops rose and 3 drops orange to a bath. Use the same combination in 10 ml carrier oil for a massage afterwards.

Pure rose oil trickled into a bath releases an amazing fragrance, which can relieve stress almost instantly.

Roman Camomile

Anthemis nobilis

Plant profile: the name 'camomile' is originally from the Greek *kamaimelon,* which means 'ground apple'. This derives from the fact that the camomile plant is low-growing and smells strongly of apples. In its non-flowering variety, this species of camomile is often used to make a fragrant lawn. The flowers, however, are required for distillation.

The oil has a pale blue colour due to the presence of a substance known as 'azulene', which has anti-inflammatory properties. The oil is now cultivated successfully in the UK.

Safety information: no issues.

Fragrance profile: fruity (apple-like), sweet, fresh and soft.

Main uses: soothes cuts, burns, sore, dry skin, nappy rash; eases menstrual cramps, premenstrual low energy and tension; soothes headaches, migraine; helps insomnia, nervous exhaustion, tension, restlessness and stress-related problems.

The yellow flowers and leaves of roman camomile are very aromatic.

Suggested blends: for skin problems, add 3 drops roman camomile, 4 drops lavender and 3 drops palmarosa to 20 ml carrier oil and apply as necessary; for baby nappy rash, use 1 drop only of camomile in 20 ml carrier oil for an extremely gentle application.

To ease menstrual symptoms, add 3 drops roman camomile and 2 drops marjoram to a warm bath, then add this combination of oils to 10 ml carrier oil and massage the lower abdomen.

For insomnia and restlessness, try vaporising 3 drops roman camomile and 3 drops lavender in the bedroom before turning in for the night.

Babies and younger children respond well to the fragrance of roman camomile essential oil.

Neroli (orange blossom)

Citrus aurantium var. amara

Plant profile: the essential oil from orange blossom is named after princess Neroli, an Italian noblewoman of the Renaissance period who perfumed her gloves with Neroli flowers. The oil has an enchanting aroma, and is costly and labour-intensive to produce, as the fragrant white flowers of the bitter orange tree have to be picked by hand. Neroli essential oil is mostly distilled in France and Morocco. Look out for pure neroli diluted in jojoba from quality essential oil ranges, as this is a more affordable way of trying this fragrance.

Safety information: no issues.

Fragrance profile: creamy-sweet, citrusy, rich and soft with green undertones.

Main uses: tones and rejuvenates the complexion, especially dry, mature or undernourished skins; helps scar tissue, wounds, cuts; eases nervous indigestion and irritable bowel symptoms; helps calm panic, shock and sudden emotional upsets.

Suggested blends: for skincare, add 3 drops neroli, 4 drops frankincense and 3 drops

Each orange blossom has to be picked by hand, making neroli – along with rose – one of the more expensive essential oils.

patchouli to 20 ml jojoba for a nourishing facial massage oil.

To heal damaged skin, add 3 drops neroli, 4 drops lavender and 4 drops myrrh to 20 ml carrier oil and apply to the area twice daily.

For nervous indigestion, add 4 drops neroli, 3 drops peppermint and 3 drops ginger to 20 ml carrier oil for gentle abdominal massage whenever necessary.

To help shock and panic, simply place 2 drops neroli on a tissue and inhale the fragrance until calm is restored.

Berry and Seed Oils

These are aromatic packages of pungent fragrance, often designed to attract animals and birds. They ingest the seeds and then eventually release them into the earth, helping plant reproduction.

Nutmeg
Myristica fragrans

Aromatic nutmegs have a spicy, cheering fragrance. They can be used in cakes and biscuits to give a distinctive flavour.

Plant profile: the nutmeg tree grows in Indonesia and Sri Lanka. The fruits are covered with a layer called mace, which is removed before processing. The highly aromatic nutmegs are steam-distilled to give a fragrant essential oil. In Western herbal tradition, nutmegs were prized for their digestive tonic and muscle-warming properties. In medieval times they were so valuable they were kept locked away.

Safety information: a strong oil, so should be used in moderation.

Fragrance profile: warm, sharp, spicy and sweet with a distinctive softness later.

Main uses: eases muscular aches and pains, arthritic pain and cold extremities; soothes and calms indigestion, stomach cramps, nausea; helps to re-energise the body after illness, speeding convalescence, uplifting the spirits and restoring the circulation.

Suggested blends: for aches and pains, add 2 drops nutmeg, 4 drops cardamom and 4 drops grapefruit to 20 ml carrier oil and massage into the affected area. To soothe the digestion, add 2 drops nutmeg, 4 drops peppermint and 4 drops ginger to 20 ml carrier oil for abdominal massage. As a restoring tonic, add 1 drop nutmeg, 2 drops black pepper and 2 drops orange to a warm bath and relax in the water. Add the same oils to 10 ml carrier oil and massage into the skin afterwards.

Blends made using nutmeg can ease muscular cramps.

Black Pepper

Piper nigrum

Plant profile: this plant is a trailing vinelike climber with lovely, heart-shaped, dark green leaves and clusters of white flowers that become the berries – or peppercorns. These turn from red to black as they mature (white pepper has had the outer layer removed). Black peppercorns are steam-distilled to yield the essential oil. The tropical plant is native to India, and the oil is produced there as well as in Indonesia and Malaysia.

Safety information: no issues.

Fragrance profile: warm, musty, sharp and spicy, with heavier sweet notes later.

Main uses: warms and stimulates blood circulation; helps to ease aches and pains; soothes indigestion, stomach cramps and constipation; strengthens the immune system, especially against influenza.

Suggested blends: to help stimulate poor or sluggish circulation, add 4 drops black pepper, 2 drops lemongrass and 4 drops cardamom to 20 ml carrier oil and massage into the affected area as needed.

Black peppercorns yield a warm and pungent oil, which has a very spicy aroma. Black pepper essential oil can boost the immune system and ease indigestion.

To help ease indigestion or constipation, add 3 drops black pepper, 3 drops peppermint and 4 drops neroli to 20 ml carrier oil and massage the abdomen twice daily.

As a tonic for the immune system, add 1 drop black pepper, 2 drops tea tree and 2 drops bergamot to a warm evening bath and soak for at least 20 minutes. Add the same oils to 20 ml carrier oil and massage the chest area afterwards.

Poor circulation can be helped by vigorously massaging the area in question with the pepper blend.

Cardamom
Elettaria cardamomum

Essential oils like cardamom improve the mood and warm the affected areas. Cardamom is a good energy tonic too.

Plant profile: a member of the same plant family as ginger, cardamom produces aromatic flowers that turn into little seed pods filled with tiny black seeds. The pods are traditionally chewed in India to sweeten the breath after eating spicy food, and the wonderful aroma of cardamom is also used to flavour Indian ice cream and confectionery. Cardamom is commonly used in Eastern medicinal traditions as a lung tonic and immunity-boosting plant remedy.

Safety information: no issues.

Fragrance profile: warm, fruity, sweet and spicy with a mouthwatering pungent freshness.

Main uses: soothes and opens the chest, helping breathing and congestion; warms and soothes stomach cramps and indigestion; uplifts the mind and gives a positive feeling when energy is low.

Suggested blends: to improve breathing, add 3 drops cardamom and 2 drops cedarwood to a bowl of nearly boiling water and inhale the vapour, repeating twice daily; add the same oils to 10 ml carrier oil and massage the chest area afterwards.

To help ease digestion problems, massage the abdomen twice daily with 3 drops cardamom, 3 drops coriander and 4 drops orange in 20 ml carrier oil.

As a tonic to raise low spirits, add 3 drops cardamom and 2 drops mandarin to a warm bath and relax in the water. Add the same oils to 10 ml carrier oil and massage into the skin afterwards.

May Chang

Litsea cubeba

May chang has berries that smell like lemon sherbert! It is not a suitable oil for babies and young children.

Plant profile: a tree from China with delicate leaves and little whitish-yellow flowers that become highly lemon-scented tiny fruits. The oil from the berries of the may chang tree is used a great deal in China as a mood enhancer and as a tonic to the heart; it calms and regulates the heart rhythm when used in massage. It is similar to lemongrass, but has a much lighter and sweeter fragrance.

Fresh lemony scents, such as may chang, have a cheering effect on the body and mind and can help ease mood swings.

Safety information: avoid using this oil on sensitive or damaged skin. It is not suitable for babies or children. Always dilute this oil, even if you are using it in the bath.

Fragrance profile: soft, sweet and fruity with a strong 'lemon sherbert' aroma that is zesty and mouthwatering.

Main uses: eases muscular aches and pains, strains and backache; eases panic or stress attacks; uplifts depression and anxiety, mood swings and tearfulness.

Suggested blends: for aches and pains, add 2 drops may chang, 4 drops juniper and 4 drops lavender and massage affected areas.

Panic and stress attacks can be eased by simply placing 2 drops may chang on a tissue and inhaling the aroma for a few minutes. Add 2 drops may chang and 3 drops neroli to a warm bath and relax in the water to recover.

Uplift moods and ease depression by massaging the body with a blend of 2 drops may chang, 2 drops rose and 6 drops frankincense in 20 ml carrier oil.

Juniper

Juniperus communis

Blue-black juniper berries are sharp and pungently scented. They take up to two years to turn black.

Plant profile: juniper is a vigorous shrub with dark green spiky leaves. The essential oil comes mainly from Germany, where the plant grows well, and also from parts of Croatia. The berries on the juniper bush take up to two years to turn black and produce the best-quality oil. Juniper is also used in making gin, and in northern European cooking it is used to give pungent flavour to root vegetables. In herbal medicine, juniper is considered to be a strong diuretic and internal cleanser.

Safety information: this is best avoided during pregnancy, and also by people with any serious kidney complaints.

Fragrance profile: pungent, peppery and camphoraceous, with sweeter, softer notes developing later.

Main uses: helps to clear lymphatic congestion and detoxify the system; opens the chest and eases breathing in respiratory complaints; freshens the mind and helps improve concentration.

Suggested blends: to help detoxify, add 2 drops juniper, 2 drops angelica and 6 drops grapefruit to 20 ml carrier oil for a vigorous daily massage to affected areas of the body.

To help respiratory complaints, add 2 drops juniper and 3 drops eucalyptus to a bowl of nearly boiling water and inhale the vapours. Do this twice daily.

To help concentration, vaporise 3 drops juniper and 3 drops lemon in a room; this also helps to clear the atmosphere and neutralise any stale or unpleasant odours.

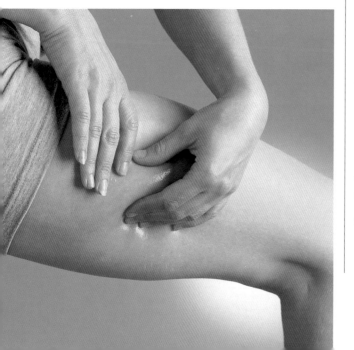

Massage blends with juniper can help improve areas of poor circulation in the legs. A vigorous daily massage is recommended.

Coriander Seed

Coriandrum sativum

Plant profile: the coriander plant is a highly aromatic herb with deliciously flavoured dark green leaves. It is easy to grow in the garden and makes a pungent addition to salad greens and a wonderful garnish for Indian dishes. The coriander plant produces umbels – umbrella-like stalks topped with little white flowers that eventually turn to brownish-coloured aromatic seeds. These are distilled to produce the essential oil in Eastern European countries, including Russia and Croatia.

Safety information: no issues.

Fragrance profile: woody, spicy and sweet with a slight hint of musk.

Main uses: warms and soothes muscular stiffness and aching joints; helps build immunity, especially in the case of influenza; eases mental exhaustion and overstretched nerves.

Coriander is a herb widely used in cooking and herbalism. It has attractive heads of white flowers.

Coriander seeds are a pungent spice and are used frequently in Indian cuisine. The leaves are also used as a delicious garnish.

Suggested blends: to warm muscles, add 3 drops coriander, 3 drops black pepper and 4 drops ginger to 20 ml carrier oil and massage twice daily. To help boost the immune system, add 2 drops coriander and 3 drops lemon to a bath; add the same oils to 10 ml carrier oil afterwards and massage into the chest area.

To ease exhaustion, add 2 drops coriander, 1 drop neroli and 2 drops lavender to a bath; the same oils can be added to 10 ml carrier oil afterwards for a massage. This routine can also help improve the quality of sleep.

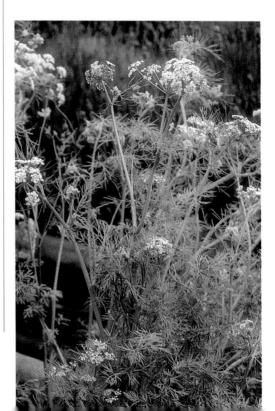

Fruit Oils

These oils are packed into tiny fragrant globules in the rind of citrus fruit. Fresh and zesty, they are mouthwatering aromas, loved by adults and children.

Orange (sweet)
Citrus sinensis

Plant profile: most orange essential oil that is commercially available is from the sweet orange tree, which originated in China. The essential oil is expressed, or crushed out of the rind of the fruit. The bitter orange tree (*Citrus aurantium*) produces petitgrain and neroli essential oils.

Orange trees are covered with delicious-smelling leaves, flowers and fruits. Orange essential oil is popular with young and old alike.

Safety information: very mildly phototoxic; avoid exposure to strong sunlight or a sunbed for 12 hours after skin application.

Fragrance profile: sweet, warm, fresh and citrusy.

Main uses: soothes stomach cramps and indigestion (especially in children); rejuvenates congested and slack skin; uplifts depression, mood swings, anxiety and emotional stress.

Children particularly love the sweet soft aroma of orange essential oil. It is a popular Christmas smell!

Suggested blends: for stomach problems, add 4 drops orange, 2 drops peppermint and 4 drops ginger to 20 ml carrier oil and massage the abdomen 2–3 times daily (halve the number of drops in 20 ml for children).

To rejuvenate tired skin, add 4 drops orange, 4 drops frankincense and 2 drops cypress to 20 ml jojoba.

To ease anxiety, add 2 drops orange, 1 drop rose and 2 drops sandalwood to a bath; use this blend in 10 ml carrier oil for massage.

Lemon

Citrus limonum

Lemon rind is packed full of fresh and zesty essential oil. It is a good oil to assist concentration and sharpen the mind.

Plant profile: the finest essential oil of lemon is considered to come from trees grown in Sicily, although the fruit is also cultivated in California, Florida and Israel. The evergreen tree is thorny and has shiny, dark green, aromatic leaves that produce an essential oil called *petitgrain citronnier*. The fragrant flowers turn into the fruit, which when ripe are a warm golden yellow. Essential oil of lemon is expressed, or squeezed out of the peel of the fruit.

Safety information: mildly phototoxic; avoid any exposure to strong sunlight or a sunbed for at least 12 hours after application of the oil to the skin.

Fragrance profile: green, citrusy and fresh, zesty and bright; softer and more sherbety tones develop with time.

Main uses: helps build immunity against colds, influenza and other viral infections; detoxifies the system and assists lymphatic drainage; freshens the mind and helps to improve concentration.

Lemon trees grow all over the Mediterranean, and particularly in Sicily. They are a wonderful sight in the summer.

Suggested blends: to help boost the immune system, vaporise 3 drops lemon and 2 drops tea tree in a room to disinfect the air; add the same oils to 10 ml carrier oil to massage the chest area twice daily.

To help detoxify the body, add 4 drops lemon, 2 drops angelica and 4 drops juniper to 20 ml carrier oil and massage the legs and other affected areas twice daily.

To assist concentration and improve alertness, add 3 drops lemon and 3 drops rosemary to a vaporiser; this is especially helpful when studying.

Mandarin

Citrus reticulata

Mandarin has a soft, bittersweet citrus aroma. The essential oil is used in soaps and cosmetics.

Plant profile: this small citrus tree is evergreen and its fruit has an immediate association with Christmas. The fruit and the expressed oil are produced mainly in Brazil, Spain and Italy. Because it is so mild and pleasant, mandarin is used as a flavouring in many confectionery items, liqueurs and soft drinks, as well as in soaps, toiletries and perfumes. It is a favourite with children.

Safety information: very mildly phototoxic; avoid exposure to strong sunlight or a sunbed for 12 hours after application to the skin.

Fragrance profile: fresh, pungent and sweet with a bright citrus zest; softer and more floral tones developing with time.

Main uses: clears congested and oily skin; soothes stomach cramps and nervous indigestion (especially in children); eases insomnia, restless sleep and troubled dreams.

Suggested blends: for oily skin, add 4 drops mandarin, 3 drops cypress and 3 drops juniper to 20 ml jojoba oil and use as a cleanser and skin-soother for evening treatment.

To ease digestion problems, add 4 drops mandarin, 2 drops roman camomile and 4 drops lavender to 20 ml carrier oil and gently massage the abdomen twice daily (halve the number of drops in 20 ml for children).

To help induce restful sleep, add 3 drops mandarin and 3 drops lavender to a vaporiser.

Vaporising mandarin essential oil at night helps to improve sleep and ease any lingering anxiety.

Grapefruit

Citrus x paradisi

The large golden grapefruit produces a different aroma to its other citrus relatives.

Plant profile: grapefruit is a hybrid which may have been derived from an old variety of fruit called the shaddock. It is now cultivated extensively in Florida in its familiar golden and pink-fleshed varieties. The essential oil is expressed from the peel, and grapefruit has an aroma quite different from its citrus relatives, thanks to the presence of sharp bitter constituents that give it freshness and zest.

Safety information: mildly phototoxic; avoid exposure to strong sunlight or a sunbed for 12 hours after application to the skin.

Fragrance profile: green, bittersweet, zesty and fresh, with a soft, powdery afternote.

Main uses: helps clear toxins and improve areas of cellulite; eases the chest and breathing in colds and influenza; eases anxiety, depression and stress, helps to relieve insomnia and disturbed dreams.

Suggested blends: for detoxification purposes, first use a skin brush on dry skin to boost the circulation, then add 4 drops grapefruit, 3 drops lemon and 3 drops juniper to 20 ml carrier oil for an evening massage of the affected areas. To help relieve chest infections, add 3 drops grapefruit and 2 drops cedarwood to a bowl of nearly boiling water and inhale the vapour for 20 minutes; add the same drops to 10 ml carrier oil afterwards and massage the chest.

To ease insomnia and anxiety, add 2 drops grapefruit and 3 drops sandalwood to a warm evening bath and relax in the water; add the same drops to 10 ml carrier oil and massage the skin afterwards.

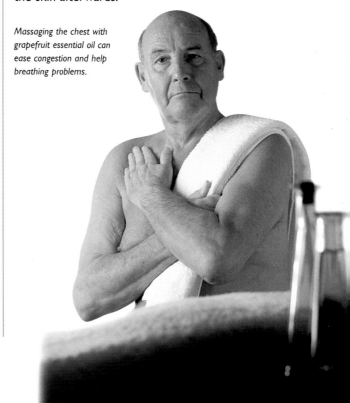

Massaging the chest with grapefruit essential oil can ease congestion and help breathing problems.

Bergamot

Citrus bergamia

Bergamot is a small and very bitter orange. It is grown in Italy, where it has been used in traditional remedies for many years.

Plant profile: bergamot is a small bitter orange grown in the Lombardy region of Italy near the town of Bergamo. The fruit has long been used in the traditional medicine of the area as a remedy for fevers and low immunity. The essential oil from the peel is best known as the flavouring of Earl Grey tea, giving the drink a fresh, citrusy flavour.

Safety information: bergamot is strongly phototoxic; avoid exposing the skin to strong sunlight or sunbeds for at least 12 hours after application. FCF (furano-coumarin free) bergamot oil is available with the phototoxic constituent removed, but the aroma of the oil is much reduced.

Fragrance profile: fresh, bright, citrusy and sweet, developing softer, rounder and warmer tones later.

Main uses: boosts immunity, helps to combat colds, influenza and respiratory complaints; eases the symptoms of vaginal thrush; soothes anxiety, depression, helps to lift low spirits and combat stress.

Suggested blends: to help boost the immune system, add 2 drops bergamot, 2 drops tea tree and 1 drop black pepper to an evening bath and relax in the water; then add the same drops of essential oil to 10 ml carrier oil and massage the chest area.

For thrush, add 2 drops bergamot and 3 drops sandalwood to a warm bath to soothe the area.

To ease stress and anxiety, vaporise 3 drops bergamot and 3 drops frankincense to create a warm and uplifting aroma.

Bergamot and tea tree oils help to improve general immunity.

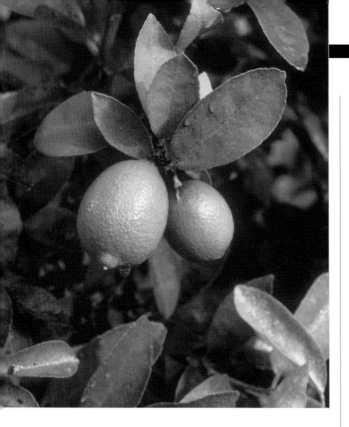

Fresh green limes are popular in Caribbean cooking. They are also an excellent source of vitamin C.

Lime

Citrus aurantifolia

Plant profile: an evergreen citrus tree, this is thorny with smooth aromatic leaves and small white flowers which turn into the fruits. Limes are about half the size of lemons and are a rich green in colour. Limes are an excellent source of vitamin C and are widely used in cookery recipes from the West Indies. The oil is expressed from the peel. The main centres of production are Florida, Cuba and Central America.

Safety information: lime is moderately phototoxic; you should avoid exposing the skin to strong sunlight or a sunbed for at least 12 hours after application.

Fragrance profile: bitter, green and fresh with a powerful zest and sharp fruity notes.

Main uses: helps detoxify and improve areas of cellulite; eases chest infections, respiratory complaints and catarrh; clears the head and improves concentration.

Suggested blends: to help detoxify, first use a skin brush to stimulate the circulation, then add 2 drops lime, 3 drops juniper and 5 drops cypress to 20 ml carrier oil and massage affected areas, as an evening treatment.

To relieve respiratory complaints, add 3 drops lime and 3 drops eucalyptus to a large bowl of nearly boiling water and inhale the vapours, twice daily for 20 minutes.

To clear the head, increase alertness and improve the atmosphere in stuffy rooms, vaporise 3 drops lime and 3 drops peppermint.

Vaporise a mixture of peppermint and lime essential oils to help improve concentration.

Simple Essential Oil Skincare

Essential oils can be used as the basis of a simple and effective skincare routine. They are particularly effective when used at night, because lying horizontally promotes an excellent supply of blood to your face, allowing maximum absorption of essential oils through the skin. Use the chart below to identify your skin type and choose the blends that will be most suitable for you.

Skin types

Normal – smooth and supple, clear in appearance, fine-textured
Dry – dull-textured, dehydrated, tends to tighten up in wind or warm temperatures
Mature – evident expression lines and slackness around eyes and mouth, less elasticity
Oily – shiny, with large obvious pores, tendency to blemishes
Combination – a greasy patch over forehead, nose and chin; dry cheek areas
Sensitive – often very pale, sensitive to sunlight and cosmetics, allergic tendency

Jojoba carrier oil is one of the best natural skin cleansers and is suitable for all types.

Cleanse

One of the best all-round skin cleansers is jojoba oil, a liquid wax from the jojoba bean. This wax is very similar to the skin's own oils, and literally dissolves dirt out of the pores. Even greasy skin can benefit, and jojoba conditions all skin types beautifully. A small amount of blend on a cotton wool pad goes a long way. Try using the cleansing blend before you get in your bath, so the steam from the bath can further open the pores before you use your toner.

Choose one of the following blends and add to 20 ml jojoba oil:

Normal/dry/mature skin: 2 drops frankincense, 4 drops sandalwood, 4 drops orange.

Oily/combination skin: 2 drops juniper, 3 drops cypress, 5 drops lemon.

Sensitive skin (half the proportions): 2 drops roman camomile, 3 drops lavender.

These blends should be used within 4 weeks. They can be kept in the fridge or at room temperature. (They last longer in the fridge.)

Tone

Good chemists, drug stores and essential oil suppliers sell floral waters, the by-products of the distillation process, which make very good toners. Use a small amount on a cotton wool pad to freshen the skin before the moisturising treatment. The following flower waters are recommended:

Normal/dry/mature skin: pure rose water or pure neroli water.

Floral waters from the distillation process make very gentle skin toners. Good chemists will stock them.

Oily/combination skin: pure lavender water.

Sensitive skin: pure camomile water or pure rose water.

Floral waters will last up to six months if kept in the fridge.

Moisturise

Night time facial treatment oils have a shelf life of about four weeks and can be made up either in sweet almond oil, recommended for dry or mature skins, or jojoba, for all skin types.

Add to 20 ml of your chosen carrier oil:

Normal/dry/mature skin: 2 drops rose, 3 drops neroli, 5 drops frankincense.

Oily/combination skin: 3 drops geranium, 3 drops cypress, 4 drops lemon.

Sensitive skin (half proportions): 3 drops roman camomile, 2 drops rose.

Massage a small amount into your face for 10 minutes, using upward strokes on your cheeks and tiny circles around your eye sockets and over your forehead. Be careful not to wipe the blend into your eyes.

Special Massage Blends

Here are some special massage blends for you to try, for physical, mood-related and seasonal reasons. They are all designed to be made up in 20 ml carrier oil, such as sweet almond, jojoba or grapeseed, a lighter and less greasy base oil. They all have a four-week shelf life. Massage relevant areas gently, using relaxing sweeping movements. Sometimes you may wish to work on yourself, but it can be soothing to let someone else – a close friend or partner – massage you.

Physical Tonics

Here are four blends for hard-working areas of the body which are constantly under strain.

Super muscle tone: for sports massage to energise and strengthen the muscles – 4 drops rosemary, 2 drops lemongrass and 4 drops ginger.

Barefoot bliss: a massage blend to help cool and soothe tired and aching feet after a long day – 3 drops peppermint, 3 drops black pepper and 4 drops lavender.

Chest relief: a wonderful blend for chest massage to ease respiratory problems –

Massage blends firmly into the limbs for the best effect.

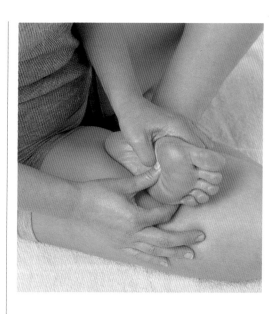

A foot massage warms and relaxes tired feet. It feels even better if someone else does it for you!

3 drops cedarwood, 3 drops frankincense and 4 drops lemon.

Neck and shoulder rescue: ask a friend or your partner to massage this blend into your aching muscles – 2 drops vetiver, 3 drops ginger and 5 drops lavender.

Mood Mixtures

Here are some ideas for more subtle blends with rich aromas. You will find them useful for lifting the spirits and easing emotional stresses and strains.

Beat the blues: 3 drops orange, 4 drops grapefruit and 3 drops sandalwood makes a wonderful relaxing, uplifting and de-stressing blend for massage.

PMT reviver: at that low time in your monthly cycle, try a blend of 4 drops palmarosa, 2 drops patchouli and 4 drops bergamot for an evening massage blend.

On cloud nine: when you need to escape without a care in the world, try 4 drops grapefruit, 2 drops neroli and 4 drops cardamom for a dreamy aroma.

Tropical retreat: create an exotic mood with 2 drops ylang ylang, 4 drops mandarin and 4 drops sandalwood – this is a fruity, rich and floral feast for the senses.

Seasonal Treats

As your energies vary, you may find that you need different massage blends to pick you up at different times of the year. Massage is particularly effective after a bath, as the skin absorbs the blend better. Spending time being massaged also helps improve your sleep – when you rest like this, your whole body can restore itself and your mind can be at peace.

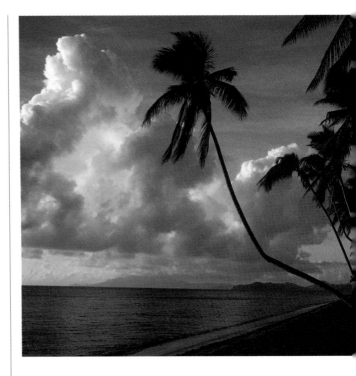

Inhale the aromas of the oils in the blends and float off into your own haven of tranquillity – a tropical beach, for example.

Springtime freshener: to help to revitalise and energise you after the long drag of wintertime – 4 drops lemon, 3 drops juniper and 3 drops peppermint.

Summer skin food: use the following blend in 20 ml jojoba oil to nourish the skin deeply – 3 drops sandalwood, 2 drops patchouli and 5 drops frankincense.

Autumn spiritual reviver: to uplift you as the nights draw in – 4 drops mandarin, 3 drops may chang and 3 drops coriander.

Winter energiser: for aches, stiffness and low vitality – 2 drops vetiver, 3 drops lemongrass and 5 drops nutmeg.

Essential Oils in Everyday Life

Essential oils are a wonderful and natural way to keep your environment fresh and to raise your energy levels. They are very portable and can easily be adapted to suit different locations and needs. Here are some ideas for using oils simply and effectively.

Home

In your home, essential oils help to personalise your living space.

Be careful to add the right number of drops of essential oil to your blends. This is important when blending for children.

Kitchen

This is one of the most frequently used and also most potentially accident-prone areas. Always keep lavender and tea tree to hand – you can use either oil neat for cuts, burns, scalds and other mishaps (put 2 drops on a cotton wool pad). A kitchen spray to remove stale odours and freshen work surfaces at the end of a day can be made in a pump-action spray bottle filled with 100 ml water, 10 drops peppermint and 15 drops lemon. Shake the bottle and spray mist into the air, or spray surfaces and wipe them down.

A pump-action spray bottle helps to spread essential oils over a much wider area.

Dining room

A vaporiser adds atmosphere to a dinner party. For example, a Christmas gathering can be fragranced with 3 drops mandarin and 3 drops nutmeg, or a summer party with 3 drops may chang and 3 drops orange. One dose of essential oils in a vaporiser will last up to 2 hours.

Living room

Again, a vaporiser can clear the atmosphere, neutralise pet odours and freshen the air. A combination like 3 drops tea tree and 3 drops lemon helps if someone has a cold or influenza. After a party the night before, 3 drops peppermint and 3 drops rosemary is very uplifting and refreshing.

Child's bedroom

An electric vaporiser is recommended for safety reasons. Essential oils can really help sleep. Add 3 drops lavender and 3 drops orange for a soothing aroma; or 3 drops lavender and 3 drops eucalyptus if there are chest problems. Try to start the vaporiser at least 10 minutes before your child goes to bed – this spreads the fragrance into the room as they fall asleep.

Travel

Essential oils can help you on the move.

Car

Vaporisers are available that plug into the cigarette lighter socket, or you can put oils on a tissue. On long journeys, 3 drops peppermint and 3 drops rosemary will help you stay alert.

Keep a tissue in your pocket when on long journeys – you can inhale oils from it when you have a break.

Vaporising oils in a bedroom will improve the quality of sleep and scent the room delightfully as well.

Trains and planes

Carry one or two essential oils with you and put a few drops onto a tissue to inhale. Lavender will help you relax, peppermint and rosemary will wake you up, and lemon or tea tree will help ease sinus congestion.

Buying and Storing Essential Oils

Here are some simple guidelines to follow to help you get the best out of your essential oil collection.

Buying Oils

There are many essential oil suppliers now selling to the public, and there is, unfortunately, a huge variation in the quality and therapeutic effectiveness of the oils available. True essential oils are not just a manufactured product, they are produced year by year and harvests can be affected by many environmental changes. Cheap essential oils are much more likely to be synthetic copies than the genuine article. Check that your supplier sources oils directly from growers.

You need to buy your oils in dark glass bottles to protect them from UV light. Oils should also have a drop dispenser in the neck of the bottle to release one drop at a time to help you calculate your blends. This is also an important safety feature: open-necked bottles

Many plants are expensive to harvest and these oils can be costly to buy. However, their divine scent makes it all worthwhile!

are a risk to children, who may swallow the contents. In any case, keep all essential oils well out of children's reach.

Storing Oils

Essential oils degrade with time. Their constituents oxidise and become unstable, smelling rancid. The cooler and more tightly closed they are kept, the longer the shelf life. How long you keep your oils depends on the storage temperature: in the fridge, most oils last up to two years, citrus oils one year.

Dark glass bottles with integrated stoppers or drop dispensers are vital if you are planning to use a lot of essential oils.

Always keep essential oils cool and out of direct sunlight. They also keep well in the fridge.

At room temperature, most oils last up to one year, citrus oils six months. The shelf life is calculated from the first day you open a new bottle. Write a date on the label or place a sticker on the bottle to remind you of the use-by date. If you are keeping oils in the fridge, you are advised to put them in an airtight box first to stop the fragrances spreading to your milk and dairy products! Out of the fridge, keep the oils tightly closed, in the dark and in a cool place. Do not use essential oils once they have gone past their shelf life, because they are then more likely to cause skin reactions.

Keeping essential oils in the fridge extends their shelf life. Make sure that the bottles are airtight at all times.

Recommended Suppliers

The following suppliers do mail order and sell high-quality ranges of essential oils.

Aromatherapy Products Ltd (suppliers of the Tisserand range, selling to 30 countries) Newtown Road, Hove, East Sussex BN3 7BA, UK
Tel: +44 (0)1273 325666;
Fax: +44 (0)1273 208444
Call them for your nearest stockist or mail order enquiries.

Essentially Oils Ltd
8–10 Mount Farm, Junction Road, Chipping Norton, Oxfordshire OX7 6NP, UK
Tel: +44 (0)1608 659544;
Fax: +44 (0)1608 659566
www.essentiallyoils.com
email: sales@essentiallyoils.com
Mail order enquiries welcome.

In the USA you are recommended to contact **National Association for Holistic Aromatherapy (NAHA)** for details of suppliers: 2000 2nd Avenue, Suite 206, Seattle WA 98121, USA
Tel: +001 (206) 2560741
www.naha.org

Glossary

Camphoraceous note
a medicinal and sharp aroma, such as marjoram.

Carrier oil
a vegetable oil used to dilute essential oils.

Cellulite
waterlogged fatty tissue deposits, particularly on thighs.

Citrus note
fresh and fruity aroma like citrus fruit.

Constituent
a fragrance ingredient of an essential oil (most oils contain up to 150).

Detoxifying
assists in the removal of toxins from the system.

Distillation
extraction of essential oils through steam followed by condensation.

Drop dispenser
a mechanism in the neck of a bottle to dispense one drop of oil.

Expression
pressing essential oils out of citrus fruit peel.

Floral note
a sweet flowery fragrance, such as rose.

Floral water
the by-product of distillation, delicately fragranced, very mild on the skin.

Inhalation
breathing in essential oil molecules to clear the chest.

Photosynthesis
plant process of sugar production using sunlight.

Phototoxic
causing skin reactions in sunlight.

Pungent note
a warm and sometimes spicy aroma.

Sensitive skin
delicate, allergy-prone skin with a tendency to rashes.

Shelf life
the length of time an essential oil can be kept before it degrades.

Solvent extraction
fragrance extraction using chemical solvents.

Synthetic fragrance
an aroma created by artificial chemicals.

Vaporiser
a unit designed to spread the fragrance of essential oils into a room.

Useful Addresses and Websites

United Kingdom

International Federation of Aromatherapists (IFA)

Stamford House, 2/4 Chiswick High Road,
London W4 1TH, UK
Tel: +44 (0)20 8742 2605

International Society of Professional Aromatherapists (ISPA)

ISPA House, 82 Ashby Road, Hinckley,
Leicestershire LE10 1SN, UK
Tel: +44 (0)1455 637987

Register of Qualified Aromatherapists (RQA)

PO BOX 3431, Danbury, Chelmsford, Essex
CM3 4UA, UK

N.B. In 2002, these three organisations are intending to amalgamate as one body called the International Federation of Professional Aromatherapists (IFPA).

USA

American Alliance of Aromatherapy

PO BOX 750428, Petaluma, CA 94975, USA
Tel: +001 (707) 778 6762

National Association for Holistic Aromatherapy (NAHA)

2000 2nd Avenue, Suite 206, Seattle WA 98121
USA
Tel: +001 (206) 265 0741
www.naha.org

Australia

International Federation of Aromatherapists

PO Box 2210, Central Park, Victoria 3145,
Australia
Tel. +0061 1902 240 125

Index